What I Wish I Would Have Known Before I Started:

Your Guide to Choosing a Gym or Program

By Aaron Nash

What I Wish I Would Have Known Before I Started:
Your Guide to Choosing a Gym or Program

All Rights Reserved

ISBN: 9781092846714

Imprint: Independently published

Cover design by Sooraj Mathew

Edited by Hilary Jastram

Resources

On the Web:

Aaron Nash – Coach

www.realplatinumfitness.com

Locations:

Platinum Fitness College Parkway

8595 College Pkway Unit 190
Fort Myers, Florida 33919

(239) 839-8749

Platinum Fitness Cape Coral

2612 Santa Barbara Bld
Cape Coral, Florida 33914

(239) 823-7282

Platinum Fitness Gulf Coast

9961 Interstate Commerce Drive Suite 100
Fort Myers, Florida 33913

(239) 839-7365

To our amazing clients who deserve to be told the truth about the fitness industry.

Table of Contents

Introduction

I wrote this book to address the top struggles and issues of clients in the fitness industry. Over the course of my career, many people have told me that they wished they'd had more knowledge on day one about the level of commitment needed when they'd joined the gym. My goal and the goal of every employee in my gym is to educate the general public on common struggles and solutions before investing hundreds and even thousands of hours into their health and fitness.

What I Wish I Would Have Known Before I Started: Your Guide to Choosing a Gym or Program will cover the major contributing factors of success in program selection and in the core areas of improving your fitness. When you are finished reading this book, you will be able to pick the program that will give you the fastest, most effective results and the highest value.

Practical examples and approaches to solving problems are provided for you. I have also included the questions you need to have answered before you ever take your wallet out to invest in another program. Gone are the days of purchasing a program that promises resolution in one area of your life, but delivers another—or worse yet, that never delivers.

I have always thought it sickening that the fitness industry seems to be the only industry allowed to make massive promises and deliver no results without any ramifications. Yes, the responsibility to do the work is the client's, especially in the health and fitness categories. But before you even get started, you need to ensure that the program you select will give you the proper tools to accomplish your goals.

Every single gym has a responsibility to clients. We all only get one body, and we need to maximize its longevity, vitality, happiness, and performance. Whatever program you select I hope you make an educated decision and ask the hard questions before investing in yourself. I use the word investment because that is exactly what your health and fitness are—an investment into a longer life and a healthier future.

Whatever you choose, whether you go to the gym or not, you're making an investment either way. If you choose to do nothing and don't exercise and improve your health and nutrition, you are investing in a lower quality of life, and disease, greater heart attack risk, injury sensitivity, joint pain, and back problems. Of course, when you neglect your body's needs, the list goes on and on and on. Never forget that a lack of investment *is* an investment into more serious problems that are associated with not taking the best care of yourself possible.

This book has been arranged in five sections; each labeled to help you quickly and easily resolve the most common problems we see in the gym—whether that is overcoming the fear to join and ask for information, structuring your program, and anything in between.

*What I Wish I Would Have Known Before I Started: Your Guide to Choosing a Gym or Program i*s your guide to choosing what's best for you so you can go on to live your healthiest life.

Section1: Getting Started

Chapter 1: Why You Need to Research Your Gym

So many fitness businesses and influencers use the same claims when talking to clients and reassuring them how much they can help them. As experts in this industry, we have heard all the BS other trainers say about losing weight and strengthening your body. More than anything, Platinum Fitness was started to help people become their best selves because I know what it feels like to want help and not get it. I also know what it feels like to want help and then have another person reach out and give you what you have wanted. False claims appear in advertisements all over the place. We hear how you can eat what you want as long as you take a particular supplement, or that you can take shortcuts to better health. Listening to this garbage, this is *harmful* to people is honestly the MOST frustrating part working with our clients. It's no fault of their own, but a majority of clients come into their first session with preconceived notions about why they can't lose weight. We set them straight before they even sit down at a single machine, pick up a free weight, or join a fitness class.

So many have been advised incorrectly, and they haven't been prepared to start the work it takes to truly transform. I don't want to scare you, but of course, building up your body and improving your health takes work!

One thing that has truly helped our clients is when they learn just how much our group personal training program entails. In case that name is as clear as mud, let me elaborate.

When we say you will benefit from group personal training, we don't mean one person walks around and prays you don't get hurt, or that we lump you in with other clients without your consent as a trainer oversees you all. In our group personal training program, there are 3-4 trainers on every session to maximize your workout every single day. These trainers are highly educated, and all of our workouts are programmed by our Doctor of Physical Therapy to ensure the workout is effective, balanced, and appropriate for any level of fitness.

When we say we are the best and get you the fastest results, it is because we have documentation to back up those claims. In the first 26 months of business, our clients' weight losses added up to over 60,000 lbs. We have never lost a "Best of" award since our business opened. We have received awards for leadership, core values, and training results from Gulfshore Life, Naples Herald, The Rotary Club, LUX, and The United Way. How do we prove it? By making it know and sharing the results with you. Our walls are covered with 18x24 posters explaining and showing the results and journeys of these amazing clients of all shapes and sizes. You can read these larger-than-life testimonials at any time in our gym. Our Doctor of Nutrition signs off on all of our nutritional programs to make sure they are safe, effective, and on the cutting edge of our industry.

When we say we hold you accountable, we actually mean it. During your 21-day trial, you are assigned multiple coaches who check in with you each week. Our GM will reach out to you to make sure you are receiving the attention you need and that you don't have any questions or concerns. You will schedule an InBody appointment to determine your body composition analysis on our state-of-the-art Body Composition Analyzer machine so we can show you exactly the state of health you are in and what areas we can help you improve on.

If you elect to take part in our 6-week challenge program, you will turn in weekly reports and weigh and measure yourself each week. You will answer multiple questions to give your coach an overview of your week and how you rated on your fitness goals. Our coaches can make changes and suggestions, or help you overcome any obstacles you may face.

You program your coaching. Meaning you can utilize our coaches as little or as much as you'd like in any of our programs. We want you to understand what to expect from us. We are dedicated to educating you and pledge to be completely transparent through every step of your health improvement process. Should you decide to trust us with your health and fitness, we will hold ourselves accountable and deliver on our promises.

It is important to read reviews, listen to testimonials, and ask your friends before you take the final step and sign your contract. Every gym should give you access to learn about their staff credentials and ask about results.

My staff and I have found that these three questions do a great job of clarifying what you really want and need in a gym:

1. What do they offer that the other gyms do not?
2. Will the gym's schedule work with your busy life?

Most importantly...

3. Do the gym's staff care about what you are trying to achieve and are they going to help you to meet your goals?

If we weren't so dedicated to our clients' results, and we hadn't celebrated these results firsthand, we wouldn't give you a 200% money back guarantee on our programs. In short, we want to remove any risk to you. Allow me to explain: If you follow our plans, make the modifications needed to continue your progress, and still don't get results, we will refund DOUBLE your money back for wasting your time. Our commitment to accountability ensures we will do right by you. We know good business equals over-delivering and exceeding expectations.

And we aim for that objective every day.

Stop wasting your time and spinning your wheels being frustrated and discouraged. Take your time to do the research you need and to ask any and all questions. An effective gym will answer your questions with proof and systems as well as documents they use to help you facilitate achieving your goals. A "talker" gym will continue to lie on social media and confuse the masses.

You have to weed through the mud to find the treasures. That is how life is today. Take your time; do your research and make the right decision. You will never regret being so invested in your health, and as you take on the fittest shape of your life, your reinvigorated body will thank you!

Chapter 2: Getting Started in the Gym

Your "Why"

When you join a gym, it is time to answer the question—*why I am doing this*? It is important to identify this reason because this is not only what gets everyone into the gym, but it's what's going to keep you moving forward during the tough times. This "why" will get you out of bed in the morning and to your workout. It is going to get you back at it when you are still sore from the previous workout. It's what's going to keep you from quitting two days, two weeks, two months, and two years down the road.

Once you determine the "why," it is time to set goals. We will help you as you make the moves to get you to your result. Envision the path you will take as a trail map that you can follow to take you where you have always dreamed of going. Your goals should be specific, measurable, actionable, realistic, and time restricted. There is a big difference between saying, "I want to lose some weight before summer," and, "I want to lose 20 lbs. by the first of June," and, "I'm going to lose 20 lbs. by going to the gym three times a week for 30 minutes a day."

How many times have we set unrealistic goals only to waste time and be sent back to where we started? Research what you're thinking about doing, or better yet, ask someone who is experienced with what you're trying to accomplish to help you come up with a reasonable and achievable plan.

Yes, this is where our trainers come in!

Not to mention the fact that Platinum Fitness employs the services of a Doctor of Physical Therapy, a Doctor of Nutrition, and a full staff of certified Fitness and Nutrition Coaches. Any one of whom can perform body composition tests, nutrition coaching, and one-on-one goal setting sessions. Platinum Fitness provides accountability combined with customized workouts designed for any fitness level, and our schedule accommodates the busiest of professionals.

Platinum Fitness is more than a gym; it is a family that provides a full-time support structure created by other members and staff. Many of the people dedicated to helping you began their fitness journeys right where you are now. Once you join Platinum Fitness failure will not be an option—but a choice.

Your "Where"

"Where do I even start?" is one of the most asked questions that people wonder about themselves when deciding they want a change in your life. You might be asking yourself that very same thing. I know because I went through the questioning cycle a thousand times as I was preparing to start the journey to a better, healthier, more fit me. Beginning any journey is intimidating, let alone one that is health and fitness related. The good news is with the proper information and preparation achieving your highest state of health doesn't have to be complicated.

Deciding to take control of your fitness and health is a big step. You have to do your homework and ask yourself some important questions. You have to be honest with yourself and make a 100% commitment to your journey, or you will fall off the wagon and give up. It's important to note that you might fall off the wagon. It's happened before with people embarking on this new path, and it will happen again. We are here to help you get back on that wagon and work with you so that little slip won't turn into a slide.

Make sure you write down the goals that you want to achieve as you consider getting fit. Written words are yet another powerful tool of accountability, but I am also a big fan of putting what you want and need out into the universe. When you declare an intention, you are more likely to follow through with the steps you need to take. On those days when your get-up-and-go gets up and leaves, seeing a reminder of the promises you made to yourself make you more apt to follow through.

Start with goals that are easy to achieve. For example, "Go to the gym three days this week" could be your first aim. When you reach that objective, mark it off and set another one. Meeting your goals, even easier ones, helps keep you motivated, and gives you the confidence to keep going. Another good thing to do to help keep you motivated is to take pictures of yourself periodically to track your progress. When your motivation starts to slip, look at those photos to help you stay focused and to reinforce in your mind that you are making progress.

One of the most important starting points in your physical fitness resolution is creating your morning routine. Morning routines can be challenging for some, but as is the case with any other habit you have to take action consistently for a period of time before you start to see lasting change in your life. Planning your routine can be a challenge as most people do not like change and have a hard time scheduling their day. Your plan needs to be realistic, and flexible. Make sure to look ahead at your week and take every day into account. For example, if you have regular plans on Wednesday morning and don't plan accordingly to move your workout, chances are you won't get that Wednesday workout in. That will throw off your plan, and also hinder you in reaching your goals.

Most importantly, remember that you will have good and bad days. You will have wins and failures, just like everyone else. But you can't let these setbacks stop you from reaching your goals. Surround yourself with a great support team that you can lean on when things get hard, and you feel like giving up. Never forget your "why," or your "where," so when life gets difficult you can redirect your focus.

If you follow the steps outlined in this section to get started, before you know it, you'll be crushing your goals again.

Section 2: Overcoming Fear

Chapter 3: Everyone Feels Intimidation

Each one of us has had moments in our life where we have been stopped in our footsteps. We've felt panicked, and nervous. We've lost our voices, and our fingers have gone numb. We've tried to scream at the top of our lungs, but nothing came out. When we've tried to move, a gravity-like force held us back.

This is what being intimidated feels like.

Intimidation happens when one is scared or lacks confidence in themselves to tackle speaking to another person (celebrity), trying a new activity that seems complicated (making a gourmet meal from scratch), and even when attempting to adopt a new mindset (abundance). Intimidation can affect a person no matter their situation, or who they are. It is when we feel intimidated and have all sorts of unannounced feelings that we have to choose our path and decide how we will react. One path will take us through a never-ending cycle of fear and intimidation where we won't accomplish what we really want to; the other path will lead to courage and success.

Even though we may take the path of intimidation first because it is "comfortable," and more familiar than the other path—and we have gotten used to living as an intimidated individual, we have it within ourselves to prevail over our fears and prove we can do anything. It's important to all of us to challenge ourselves to grow in this way. Choosing to push yourself when you are scared is an incredible high that only you will experience because you are the only one who knows what you are capable of. And spoiler alert: what you are capable of is a lot!

By choosing the path of overcoming intimidation, we gain strength and the ability to fight back our fears, and as we do, we show ourselves how strong we really are. When we're on the path of intimidation, we don't see the value of others because we are so consumed with worrying about the risks we might have to take. But when we are ready to take the leap of faith and go with our gut feeling—that urge we have to do more and be more, to face down what we never thought we could—we grow as people, and it shapes us for the better.

According to *Curious Mind Magazine,* these eight powerful personality traits might intimidate people, but it's also fascinating to note, these are the traits of a leader.

1. You don't need attention
2. You are not concerned with pleasing everyone
3. You don't put up with excuses
4. You hate small talk

5. You can't stand ignorance and insensitivity

6. You stick to your morals

7. You admit when you're wrong

8. You are not arrogant; you have a strong attitude

As a professional in the health and fitness field and the owner of Platinum Fitness, I have observed those who have strong personalities and those who do not. Those who are continually intimidated or constantly fear strong personalities hold themselves and other people back. But those who step up and want to adapt to a more upbeat environment will beat that intimidation right down, and then they will be rewarded with the courage to accomplish more! It is very difficult to attempt to break the cycle of holding back. I have seen that this is especially hard for clients who have come from different backgrounds and family dynamics where intimidation was used as a scare tactic. When you do break the cycle, it is a feeling like no other because not only have you stopped the fear in yourself, but you have sent out a message that the way life used to be is not okay. If you want to tap into unstoppable empowerment, conquer intimidation.

When I see clients work on mindset aspects of themselves, it is beautiful. The transformations in the decisions they make and how they take care of their body is mind-blowing. Nothing makes me feel prouder or happier than to witness groups of clients who never thought they would see the end of intimidation or the fear of failing.

On multiple occasions, two groups of clients, those intimidated and those who intimidate, have come together into one melting pot. They have found common ground in the fitness world. They have created these strong bonds because they respect each other and the actions it took on each person's part to contribute to the new dynamic.

Through continuous encouragement from peers and family, the fear of intimidation can be dismissed, and become just a faint memory of all that you were afraid of once upon a time. If you are anticipating that your fears will get larger the closer you get to them, it's an awesome surprise to find out that when we confront our fears, we learn just how manageable they are.

Setting a new health and fitness goal comes with a lot of doubts and fears to overcome. One of those obstacles may arise before you even step into the gym. Gym intimidation affects almost everyone and is absolutely normal, yet it is still not an easy challenge to overcome. You may be unsure of where to start or even how to start; you may be afraid that someone is watching and judging you, or you may be afraid that you are unable to participate in a fitness program due to an injury or your level of ability. I am here to assure you that all of these reasons for being intimidated to grow yourself for the better will not be an issue at Platinum Fitness.

Our entire staff has done their best to make sure you always feel welcomed and accepted whether you are on the floor, in a class, making a meal plan or working with our doctors of fitness and nutrition.

When you first walk into a typical new gym, most people have no idea where to start. They gravitate toward the machines, usually with no idea how to use them, how many reps they should be doing, what body part they should be targeting, how long they should be working, etc. There will NEVER be a day when you come into Platinum Fitness that you have to worry about any of those obstacles. Exercise programs are put together and approved by our on-staff Doctor of Physical Therapy who ensures our clients receive the best guidance. He assures that we create programs that hit the best combination of muscle groups as they give you a challenging yet doable workout within 30-minutes. He is also there to help modify any exercises that you are unable to execute due to injury or lack of physical readiness. All the trainers on staff are experienced in modifications and are made aware of injuries before you even start your workout.

You can relax your mind when it comes to planning your diet as well. Platinum offers personalized nutrition programs that are designed for you to lose weight in a healthy and maintainable way. The nutrition plans are explained to you by a coach on staff, who will also help to hold you accountable to following the plan. The coaches at Platinum fitness only want the success and improvement of the clients they encounter. Their passion is helping people become the best versions of themselves possible. You will never feel as if you are just another number in the gym.

The clients at Platinum are attracted to the judgment-free zone that we have established in our culture. Everyone that started at Platinum has gone through the same anxieties and fears you are having, so they would never want you to feel as if they are judging. Most people who come to our facility are there because they can get in and out quickly, but also because they don't have to worry about how they look when they work out. Everyone in the room has the same aim, to get healthier and progress in their fitness plan. If you are doing an exercise wrong, a trainer will be with you immediately to explain how to do the movement properly and safely!

Our gym has built an amazing community. We call ourselves a family because we treat each other as family. In our eyes, the best families are the ones you get to choose. The ones who love you and want the best for you even if you're not blood. We say, "Family on 3!" at the end of every class because we want to remind you that even after you work out, we are still here. We will still care about you once you walk out the gym doors.

Chapter 4: Fear of Failure

The ironic thing about the fear of failure is that fear itself causes failure. What I mean by this is that so many times, we allow the motivation to *avoid* failure to exceed our motivation to succeed. It is this fear of failure that causes us to subconsciously sabotage our chances of success in a variety of ways.

In so many cases, the fear of failing can make sense, but when it comes to the gym...what can you *really* fail at? In the world of fitness, there is no one way to benchmark your success. Every single person has a different journey and different goals they want to achieve for themselves. So again, I ask the question: *How could you possibly fail?*

Let me go ahead and answer the question for you by saying, "It is IMPOSSIBLE for you to fail at fitness." The only way to fail is not to start at all.

Consider this: At the beginning of anyone's fitness journey they were not repping out 100 push-ups or squatting with the heaviest weight or even making it through an entire workout without feeling defeated. But does that mean they failed? Absolutely not, because you need to start somewhere!

Sometimes, it's hard for us to imagine ourselves as ever being successful at something we've either never done before or haven't done in a very long time. It's even harder to imagine walking into a gym, feeling completely clueless, and somehow succeeding at anything at all. At Platinum Fitness we understand that, and we also know this makes us different. The majority of people that walk through our doors have no idea what they're doing. It's OUR job to teach them.

Now, I already told you it was impossible to fail at fitness, but for those of you who didn't believe me, let me ask this: *How could you fail if there are trainers who are there to guide you through EVERY part of your fitness journey? How could you fail, if we're teaching you how to exercise, correcting your form throughout every workout, telling you exactly what to eat, what not to eat, and how much to eat, etc.* When you add in those factors, it is most definitely IMPOSSIBLE to fail.

So, if there's no way you could possibly fail, what is there to fear? Looks like I might've just solved your problem, huh? Unfortunately, that means you no longer have any excuse as to why you can't start your fitness journey right this second.

In addition to being a part of your family, we are all harmless jokesters intent on having fun and in getting you to look at your aspirations differently.

Fear of failure can stop us from living our lives to the fullest and making our dreams a reality. Fear can be paralyzing and keep you from trying. We teach children to learn from their mistakes and try again. As adults, we view failure as a negative outcome rather than a possible step toward success. But this isn't fair to view ourselves this way because just as we would consider when teaching a child something new, we cannot assume that we will be masters at something we've never done. It is important to turn our focus away from perfection and work on being a little bit better each time. How will you know if you're good at something if you don't take a risk and try? Don't let the fear of failure force you to fail. Failure is part of the process of achieving a goal.

Maybe learning a new way to regard fear will help you.

Did you know that fear is a chain reaction in the brain that starts with a stressful stimulus and ends with the release of chemicals that cause fast breathing, a racing heart, and other anxiety-related symptoms? This is known as the "fight or flight" response. The stimulus could be a snake, being alone in the dark or joining a new gym. Whether your fear is physical or emotional, it triggers the same primitive survival response. According to research at Cambridge University, memory-forming portions of the brain react simultaneously with the fear response. Your subconscious is not only planning to survive; it's learning. If your body is constantly learning, then you can teach it to respond differently. Once your fear is identified, you can learn to separate physical fear from emotional fear. Don't let emotional fear stop you from trying something new. It's only scary at first, over time, your body learns to let go of the fear.

Fear is not always a bad thing; we all feel it. Even people like successful athletes, actors and musicians have to confront it. No one is immune to it. The first day I joined a gym, I was terrified, but I pushed back the fear and didn't let that stop me. It was the best decision of my life. All I knew when I opened that gym door was that I just wanted to change, so I took a risk and went for it.

Don't forget: One decision, one choice can change your life in ways you never imagined.

You can channel the energy fear creates and fight for what you want rather than taking flight. Let go of the need to be perfect. Allow yourself to learn and grow. No one is perfect all the time. Life is not perfect all the time. As long as you're working on being a better version of you, you're winning.

The only time we fail is when we stop trying (which means we are the only force responsible for our failure).

At Platinum Fitness, we understand your fears. We are changing fitness norms and have created a positive and safe environment. We have a wide demographic of members from millennials to baby boomers that represent all fitness levels. We create our workouts to be challenging but able to fit everyone. Our family atmosphere creates a support system from both our coaches and members. We learn and grow as a family, and we are personally invested in you as an individual.

If you are contemplating starting a new fitness journey, don't let fear get in the way. It's okay to be afraid of the unknown, but it can also be exciting! Dream big and go for it. Life is long, and you want to live it to the fullest. We want that for you, too. Take a risk; and remember, you only fail when you don't try.

Section 3:
Injuries/Modifications

Chapter 5: Exercise Helps Resolve Injuries and Chronic Pain

You may not know this, but personal trainers understand your apprehension about exercising after injury or when you are experiencing pain. Maybe your knee clicks when you squat. Maybe your lower back bothers you during planks, or you might have a chronic condition that affects the exercises you can do in the gym. All of these issues—with the exception of some chronic diseases—are related to underlying movement dysfunction in the body. This means that a particular muscle group might be weakened and troubling you. You might struggle with range of motion deficits, poor alignment/form, or obesity.

Listen carefully: Not one of these issues can be improved upon by NOT exercising, by resting your body or a particular part of it, or even "giving it time." Not to mention, a lack of physical activity is one of the leading contributors to preventable health concerns worldwide. Every single one of these conditions CAN absolutely be improved with movement, strengthening, graded exercise, and focused coaching.

Platinum Fitness members have rotator cuff issues, fused limbs, replaced hips and knees, rheumatoid arthritis and low back pain and injuries. We have modified programs for clients undergoing cancer treatments, returning to sports after an injury, and we have also worked with clients post-surgery. In fact, we have never seen a client in perfect physical health.

We have worked with and helped clients just like you. What is the common theme among our clients? Movement, exercise, fitness, and nutrition has helped them to regain control over their body as it has mitigated the injury or condition primarily holding them back. Movement is medicine, and through movement, we can help you once again feel confident about your health, fitness, and wellness.

At Platinum Fitness, we proudly employ the most credentialed and educated staff of coaches in the fitness industry. Each of our coaches undergoes exercise modification training for injury prevention and the accommodation of prior injuries. Our Doctor of Physical Therapy is also the Director of Programming and ensures that all workouts are comprehensive, effective, and safe. He is available to meet with clients on a case-by-case basis to outline specific program modifications to assist them in safely meeting their fitness goals.

Our staff holds degrees in the fields of health sciences, kinesiology, strength and conditioning, and physical fitness. We are equipped to help you succeed. Your injuries and physical limitations do not define you. How you respond to your challenges, will, however, dictate your future path.

Chapter 6: Injuries, Modification, and Why Your Health and Fitness Shouldn't Suffer

Nowadays, many people are afraid to embrace a lifestyle of health and fitness. There are many reasons for this hesitation, many stemming from injuries or emotional or physical limitations. At Platinum Fitness, we know this and take ample steps and precautions to take the "fear" out of the experience for our new and/or returning clients.

I had mentioned that we have never seen a client in perfect physical health and that is because there is no such thing. Even merely acknowledging that fact helps to alleviate a nervous and self-conscious state. When you walk in our front doors, you will feel peace of mind. Everyone in your yoga or group fitness classes has some ailment. You will see the same reality on the fitness floor. All of our clients come in knowing they are going to be fully taken care of no matter their need.

At this point, you are probably wondering *well, how do you combat these types of physical obstacles in the fitness world? Who can help me?* First, our staff is highly educated, and only approves workouts that are functional and safe for the masses. These regimens are followed by every single trainer who also undergoes continuing form correction education as well as exercise modification training. Our trainers constantly stay on top of the newest research and techniques, which enables them to give the very best to our clients.

For those with the fear of joining a new gym only to be unnoticed or slip through the cracks, your worries are over. Platinum has three to four trainers on the floor at all times to ensure continuous observation and monitoring of safety and form. They are ready for any questions and to offer aid wherever it may be needed.

Having had an injury or dealing with one can be scary and nerve-wracking. It can greatly cut down one's desire, motivation, and confidence. But, be assured, there is nothing that our crew of trainers can't work around, supplement, or alter. The key to getting past both the fear and the injury itself is to work with knowledgeable professionals in a safe and secure manner. Your knees may be crunching; your hips cracking, or your shoulders popping, but don't let those noises become sounds of discouragement. The only way to make yourself feel better and help your body is through movement, exercise, and strengthening your muscles and form. We have applied the exact same idea behind physical therapy and rehabilitation to our regimens. The goal is to avoid the most inactivity and prevent most old injuries from staying in a weakened state.

A wide variety of ways to modify workouts so they can be done by anyone with any past or present injury exists. This is what we focus on. Depending on what the injury is and what limitations are presented we can reduce weight and the speed at which the exercise is performed; we can limit range of motion, remove the weight altogether and use your body weight as well. We can switch to resistance bands or—in very serious cases—change or eliminate an entire exercise if need be.

As you can see, numerous adaptations around individual limitations are possible. Working with educated and knowledgeable professionals who specialize in injury rehabilitation is a must, especially when you are just coming back to the gym or starting a fitness routine. Benefitting yourself and making improvements upon your physical well-being should not be determined or deterred due to injury. You deserve to do what you need to do to embark on self-improvement without fear or hesitation. This is why our trainers are here for you, and why we conduct our programs the way we do. Everything we recommend helps make your health and fitness goals attainable.

Section 4: Weight Loss/Nutrition

Chapter 7: A Good Support Team is Necessary for Weight Loss

Finding a support team can mean the difference between success and failure when it comes to reaching your health and fitness goals. You'll want to build your team based on the following principles in this chapter.

Weight loss can feel like a very lonely journey. Many people walk into a new gym with the goal of getting healthy but soon become overwhelmed with feelings of insecurity and doubt. Not knowing where to start or being afraid of looking foolish can stop a person before they even get started. This is where a strong support system comes in. By surrounding yourself with the people who will uplift you, you can move past the fear and doubt and move toward your personal health and fitness goals.

However, it's important to understand the different roles each person may play in your journey. Recognizing that each member of your team each supports a different need will help you to know who and when to lean on them. This knowledge of where to turn can be just as important to figure out as surrounding yourself with the right people.

Your Team Includes:

1. The Workout Partner. This person will hold you accountable for showing up and putting in the sweat equity. Most people have no problem quitting on themselves but quitting on someone else can be a hard pill to swallow. Your workout partner should be in better shape than you. They shouldn't allow you to slide by with average effort and they should push you out of your comfort zone.

2. The Realist. This person will be honest with you about the good, the bad, and the ugly. The realist won't sugarcoat facts. They are probably the most important member of your team because they will force you to be the best version of yourself in all aspects of your journey.

3. Family. Having members of your family on your team can be a double-edged sword so be careful. Spouses, children, brothers, and sisters may love you unconditionally and will be there through the ups and downs. They may also be the ones who distract and derail you the most. They will be the first ones to ask you to go out and eat, the first ones to hand you that piece of birthday cake at a party, and the last to hold you accountable when you're getting off track. Be very clear on your goals and expectations with this group. If you set

boundaries from the beginning of your journey, family can be a great support system.

4. The Coach. This person is going to create your road map to success. The greatest players and teams in the world have coaches. The coach knows how to run the play and can make the adjustments necessary to push through plateaus as he or she teaches you the habits needed for a lifetime of success. When finding a coach, do your research. These days, too many "coaches" in the fitness industry make false claims or falsify their credentials. Not all coaches are created equally. Find someone who is on the same journey as you are but who is further down the path. Before you invite them to be a part of your team ask who they have worked with. Reputation and referrals are everything.

Assembling your team is the first step. But understand that your team can't do the work for you. Without you showing up every day and putting in the work, your teammates mean nothing. Until you put forth 100% effort, no one else will either. Embrace the journey; embrace the suck. It won't be easy, but you will come out on the other side better for it.

Chapter 8: Eating for a Result

When I ask a client how they would describe their diet, the answer I usually get back is: "Oh, I eat healthy." Well, I can't begin to explain how meaningless that statement is. The term "healthy" is so overused when discussing diet that it has become completely arbitrary. If you eat "healthy," why are you gaining weight? Why are you constantly getting sick? Why can't you make it through a 30-minute workout?

It's because you aren't eating for a result.

What does it mean to eat for a result? It means that the design and structure of your diet actually push you in the direction of your goals. When we look at a well-designed, results-oriented diet, we check for improvement in these three areas:

1. Health

2. Performance

3. Body Composition

Let's break down what each of these terms means and how Platinum Fitness designs our diets to achieve results in each category.

Health. Eating for your health means exactly what you think it does. You need a nutrient-rich diet with a variety of whole foods, such as fruits, vegetables, healthy fats, and complex carbs, to cover your daily needs. Obtaining the nutrients you need from the food you eat is essential for optimizing immune function, gut health, hormone production, and so much more. Eating for your health comes down to meeting your micronutrient requirements (vitamins and minerals) as well as consuming enough water and calories each day.

Performance can reference a powerlifter squatting 800 lbs., an elite runner crushing a 2.5-hour marathon, or an 80-year-old woman being able to walk up the stairs to her bedroom at night. While micronutrients are just as important for sustaining performance as they are for health, macronutrients, your proteins, carbohydrates, and fats are also vital. Protein is essential for everyone, as it is necessary for repairing muscle and recovering—and at some point or another, each of us will find ourselves in a state of health where we need to recover from an illness or accident as well as repair any damage that has occurred in our bodies. Carbohydrates and fats, on the other hand, are your primary fuel sources and the amount that you need varies according to the individual and their lifestyle. A high-performance athlete will need more carbohydrates in their diet to meet the high-energy demands of their sports; while someone else with less demanding energy requirements will do fine with more fats and fewer carbohydrates, or any combination of the two.

Body Composition. This factor refers to increasing your muscle mass and decreasing your body fat percentage. If you want to reach a goal in this category, then calorie intake will be the primary focus. Simply put, to lose fat, you need to consume fewer calories than you burn. Period. When designing a nutrition/diet plan, we go a step further than just aiming for staying ahead of what you eat. We break down your calorie intake into protein, carbohydrates, and fats. As mentioned, protein is essential to repair and recovery as well as building muscles, while carbohydrates and fats will be used in some combination to provide fuel to sustain performance during workouts and daily tasks. Aim to achieve the optimal results with carbohydrates and fat while remaining within your daily calorie intake.

Based on your age, sex, height, weight, body fat percentage, and individual goals, we determine the number of calories you should be consuming each day, and then we break them down into the three macronutrient categories you need: protein, carbohydrates, and fats. We also provide you with a list of foods that are deemed nutrient-dense. The bonus is you get to choose which foods you eat! We will never tell you to eat a certain food; if you don't like it; don't eat it. You will be taught how to read food labels and utilize direct macro counting to hit all your target numbers and achieve the goals you deserve.

Dieting isn't easy, but it doesn't have to be complicated either. Follow the guidelines; eat for the results, and you can achieve your goals.

No matter how hard you work on exercising and working out, if you don't find a way to understand food/nutrients and utilize that understanding consistently, you will never achieve the results you seek.

It's not enough to say you're going to lose 15 lbs. because you want to and that you will do it by eating healthier.

That's simply not going to cut it.

What will cut it is eating micronutrients and macronutrients for your individual makeup, your lifestyle and health goals.

Nutrition that works and gives results is:

1. Simple
2. Intuitive
3. Unique to an individual's lifestyle

If your diet plan is too complicated, it is not sustainable long term. If it doesn't take into account your true needs, then it becomes inefficient, time-consuming, and impossible to follow for most busy individuals. Works for Sally Joe is likely not going be what works for Billy Bob.

As a coach, some of the first questions I ask a client who claims to "eat healthy" are:

1. "How much water do you drink?"—You should be consuming about half of your body weight in ounces of water per day.

2. "How is your micronutrition, or how many vitamins and minerals do you consume daily?"—Does your diet consist of a wide variety of colorful veggies and fruit that help you perform at your best? Are you "eating the rainbow" every day?

3. "How is your protein intake?"—Are you allowing your body to build and maintain muscle?

4. "Do you consume essential fatty acids consistently?" — What sources are you choosing to obtain the fat necessary for your hormone regulation, brain function, vitamin absorption, and much more?

However the client answers these questions along with a few follow up ones, usually gives me a solid gauge of how off they might be. To truly make an impact in someone's life you can't just throw arbitrary statements at people and expect you will light a fire in them that will produce a transformation. You must LISTEN to their needs and goals, LEARN how they live, FIND what inspires them, and work TOGETHER to create the right mindset and nutrition plan that's unique to their lifestyle.

That's precisely what we do here at Platinum Fitness.

After a good nutrition plan is created, you and your nutritionist must track every bit of progress. As you progress through your journey, your nutritionist should make adjustments and corrections. We teach people about food and nutrients and how to fuel their bodies to perform at the highest level possible. We find out what is holding them back and actively work with passion to change self-destructive habits.

Food is energy, but it is also information. When you eat nutrient-rich foods, which are full of information, you give your genes instructions to control your metabolism. So, depending on what/how much you consume, your metabolism translates those instructions, which results in complex metabolic signals that control your weight by either turning on or off fat-burning hormones in your body. The key to sustainable, effortless fat loss is gaining the knowledge of which foods and macro amounts send the right information to your metabolism to ignite fat burning.

There is no cookie cutter approach to nutrition. Everyone is different, has different needs, reactions, and goals that can change with any given time frame or change in circumstances. The objective is to have a healthy relationship with food, understand it as a fuel source, and learn about your body and how it adapts based on your nutritional intake and exercise. Keep things simple and stay committed to getting 1% better with nutrition every day.

Effective calorie counting will help with weight loss, but our goal for you at Platinum Fitness is not just for you to lose weight, but to have QUALITY fat loss and healthy, resilient, muscular bodies.

The key to proper nutrition and eating for results is to create routines that are sustainable. Massive changes are not replicable or even doable for most people. It's all about PREPARATION. Those who succeed in their diets do a fantastic job at planning efficiently and breaking down every meal. They understand what needs are being met and the ones that aren't. They don't beat themselves up about being over on protein one day and then let that one day cause them to spiral out of control the rest of the week. They learn, adapt and overcome by using the plan customized just for them.

We all have struggles. At Platinum, we are here to find out what is causing you to struggle and provide the empathetic support to help you build healthy habits that strengthen you. One. Simple. Step. At. A. Time.

Section 5: Mindset

Chapter 9: Creating the Right Mindset

Lately, it seems these phrases from "life coaches" are all over social media:

"Mindset is everything."

"Perception is reality."

"Strong mind, strong body."

These are absolutely true statements.

But at this moment in time maybe you feel as though you have a weak mindset. You might feel as though you don't have the discipline and mental toughness to succeed in your health and fitness goals. And although you don't necessarily need to be prepared in this way to take that first step, you will definitely need discipline and mental toughness to stay consistent and keep moving forward.

The truth is, 95% of our clients:

1. Have never worked out before
2. Haven't exercised in 10+ years
3. Have never tested themselves physically
4. Haven't set any physical standards for themselves
5. Have never reached their full fitness potential
6. Have never created healthy habits
7. Have never formed a disciplined and strong mind

Over 90% of our clients were JUST like you when they began their journey. They were scared to start. Not confident in their abilities and potential. Intimated and afraid of being judged. Broken by previous experiences. Fearful of pushing their limits. Terrified of failing.

All of these worries relate back to mindset. Because *what you are scared, nervous, or even terrified of is exactly what you really want to go after, deep down.*

Read that again.

You WANT to be a healthier individual, a stronger human (both physically and mentally). You WANT to feel confident in your appearance and abilities and to test your limits and boundaries. You WANT to play with your kids without having to stop every 20 seconds to catch your breath. You WANT to live longer to see your children graduate/get married/have kids of their own.

You WANT to stop allowing yourself to get in your own way.

You WANT to hit all of those goals, but you feel as though your mindset is holding you back.

What if I told you that we have helped THOUSANDS of individuals completely transform their mindset along with their bodies?

What if I told you that people just like you have created a massively strong foundation and reached every single goal they've ever had for themselves?

What if I told you that our family at Platinum Fitness could help you find and develop that new, and improved mindset to take you to that next level of your life?

Not only do we have the best coaches in Southwest Florida (in fact, I will confidently say in all of Florida), but we also have THE BEST members of any gym, organization, or club in America.

Our coaches are some of the most highly educated and experienced individuals you will find in the health and fitness space (that is a hiring requirement at Platinum Fitness). Each and every one of us genuinely wants to help you succeed.

Our coaches will:

- Push you.
- Encourage you.
- Hold you accountable.
- Help you overcome any obstacles. Both physical and mental.
- Help you achieve any goals that you may have for yourself.
- Help restructure your mentality to move you forward on your journey.

Beyond our coaches, we legitimately have the most encouraging, supporting, and loving members (family) of all time. Being around this family will absolutely make you a better, stronger, and more resilient human being. This family will help you create that unbreakable mindset that you need to consistently show up, and get your work done.

Our family will hold you accountable and be there for you to keep your feet moving in the right direction.

Not only will you be welcomed with the most accepting and comforting arms of all time, but you will also be pushed and encouraged to be the absolute best version of yourself, each and every day. With the combination of our amazing trainers and members, we will help you create your new mindset.

We will provide you with the tools to train your mind and your body, and the tools to completely transform the way you think, and act. We will provide a healthier approach to food, and a healthier approach to working out, growing internally, and approaching life as a whole. We will regrow, repair, and reshape your entire mindset.

You will become the person you have always dreamt of becoming.

Strong.
Resilient.
Unbreakable.

Have you heard the saying, "If you do what you've done, you will get what you've always gotten?"

A majority of people who start a new training program come with one foot in and one foot out of their program.

These clients may give a half-attempted effort and when the weight doesn't just fly off, for example, they will either pull back on their work ethic or quit altogether. In these circumstances, it is never YOU, the program or the food that isn't working.

What isn't working is that person's mindset.

Those of us with a weaker mindset already fight with thoughts of self-defeat, poor morale, and low expectations, but somewhere in our hearts we see other people living their best life in their healthiest body, and so we think *what do we have to lose?* You will put in the exact amount of work that correlates with your way of thinking. It is time to throw away those old thinking habits and embrace a change. These are the top three methods to the madness of changing your mindset.

1. Beliefs and Identity: These two pieces that are critical to your healthy mindset ties into so many areas. They not only tie into what you think of in terms of religious and scientific law, but beliefs and identity also

shape what kind of person you are, what you take offense to, and even who you *believe* you are. Study after study on identity, as well as beliefs that make up identity, have been performed. These studies found that people will act in accordance with who they believe they are. People who believe themselves to be husky or overweight will always find a way to get back to the comfort of their old lifestyles no matter how self-defeating they are. Beliefs can shape your very destiny and are a huge catalyst in composing your mindset. People can change and you can, too. It all starts with shifting your beliefs.

To change your beliefs, you must take action. If, for example, you think of yourself as lazy, then you have made being lazy a part of your identity. However, as you begin to follow through with prepping your meals and working out, you will be living a real-life example of what lazy people don't do: take action. Taking action is powerful, but most people don't take action without having a belief centered on why they need to keep going. A simple change in your beliefs can have an astonishing impact on your overall results.

2. Motivation: This is what pushes us and allows us to take action. Motivation stems from dissatisfaction with a present situation and is the base and driving force for all the hard work that you are about to put in. I've heard that people make choices for emotional reasons and justify their decisions with logic. This is why you must find your "WHY." If your goal is to lose 20 lbs. because your doctor says you need to, logically, that makes sense. Still, people drink and smoke cigarettes every day even

though they know doing so is bad for them. The logical understanding isn't enough to motivate people to make real-life changes to get to their goal. Make your motivations emotional, and you will be more likely to hit your targets.

The most motivating "why" I ever heard in all my years in the fitness industry came from a man, Steve who was 400 lbs. I asked him why he wanted to lose the weight, and he told me: "Because I am absolutely disgusted with the way I look. I don't like what I see in the mirror. I've been eating like a pig, and my body shows it. I want to be proud of who I see, and I need to make a change NOW! I also don't want to die, and if I keep this up, I am digging myself an early grave. I need your help today."

Steve lost 150 lbs. in one year. Not because he had convinced himself with logic that he needed to do it, but because the need to lose weight became emotional for him.

3. Mindset of a Champion: I've learned there are two types of mindsets. One is the growth mindset, and the other is the fixed mindset. A fixed mindset believes, "If I'm not born with it, I can't change it." We are all capable of a certain amount of success but to reach our full potential; we need to embrace the growth mindset. We need to follow the mentality that we are willing to DIE for what we believe in. Learn from failures, embrace challenges, work your ass off! We can all grow and become better, but we must be willing to put in the work every day.

Chapter 10: Accountability, Support, Character, Time

Accountability

Have you ever been punched in the mouth? No really...just popped right in the kisser? If you have, you know this feeling: the wooziness, the shock that knocks you back, the energy transferred from your head to your toes, the hit to both your body and pride, the absolute rush of adrenaline that courses through you and the wakeup call it gives you.

Being held accountable makes me think of this analogy. Hear me out. Accountability wakes you up, keeps you alert, and can knock you off your dadgum feet. It holds you to a higher standard and forces you to make the decision to make a change or get popped in the mouth again.

If you are reading this right now, it's because you either already have or are getting ready to make the decision to put your health, fitness, and life as top priorities. Before you even think about doing your first meal prep or taking your first step into a gym, you must take a few actions to ensure your success. It's easy to hype yourself up and get motivated when you are starting a new challenge. It's also just as easy to lose the fire, fade out, and end up right back where you started. This is where accountability comes in.

When you are accountable for your actions, you are required or expected to behave in a particular and understandable way that is in keeping with your goals.

Support

If you want to give yourself the greatest shot at conforming to being accountable, surround yourself with like-minded people who are willing to say what you NEED to hear whether you WANT to hear it or not.

I started this chapter by asking if you had ever been punched in the mouth. My answer to that question would be yes, and believe it or not, the majority of those times that I was clobbered in the face came from some of my best friends. They cared enough about me to shut my mouth for me when I couldn't tame my tongue. They held me to a higher standard, showed me I was better than how I was representing myself and gave me the wakeup call I needed to change. It doesn't matter if you are trying to lose weight, gain weight, burn fat, build muscle, increase athleticism, overcome an injury, or prolong functional movement; if you do not have a group of people who are going to hold you accountable, you will lose. "As iron sharpens iron, so one person sharpens another." (Proverbs 27:17.) Your accountability group should be made up of driven individuals who care about you and your well-being, who understand your goals clearly, and who are devoted enough to you to make sure when you slip up (and you will slip up), that you hear about it. This team will set the standard so high for you it will seem almost impossible to reach the expectations, but it is that standard that will drive both you and them to wake up every day and refuse ever to settle, back down, and quit. If you have "friends" who aren't willing to do that for you, then you need to reevaluate your circle.

Once you are part of such a dynamic, energetic, and honest group, you know what is expected every day. Enter support. Accountability and support are both crucial, but both different. Accountability is where motivation and expectation come in. Support is only going to come from your closest friends and family. When I reference support, I'm talking about the brother or sister who shows up at your door at 2am because you're struggling. Support is the friend who stands on the other side of the casket as you carry a loved one.

Wherever you are trying to go in your fitness journey, you are going to run into adversity. You are going to be put into situations where you are tired, sick, barely holding it together, discouraged and feeling defeated. Your support will take the form of the person you confront when you are in that condition; it's the one person who will kick down the door and go out guns blazin' to help you. The reason so many people mess up using their support system is that they are either too stubborn to allow themselves to be helped; they are too vulnerable, or the support receive is too soft to help uphold the goal. Support isn't coddling. It isn't justifying your failures with excuses. It's wiping the dirt off your shoulder and helping you get back up. Support is showing you there is always a way to fight.

If your family is your biggest support, make sure they not only know what your goals are but that they respect those goals. So, when it's a random Wednesday night, and your college team is playing a big game, they aren't shoving pizza and cheesecake in your face, convincing you "to enjoy the little things. Live your life. Celebrate the situation." In reality, that situation doesn't call for pizza. It calls for a kick in the keister and a light to illuminate your road to success. The only way to ensure that your support team defends you is by selecting people in your group wisely and letting them know, from the beginning, respectfully, to get the hell out of your space with their limiting mentality.

We've covered that you need people to hold you accountable, to set the bar high, and ensure you aren't going to quit. You need the support, so when work is busy, life is tough, and adversity smacks you so hard it feels like you kissed a freight train, you have the encouragement and love to keep going. But do you have what it takes to be successful internally?

Character

What you do when no one is looking? The decisions that you make when you are all by yourself define your character. Character is important because your accountability partner is not going to sit by the pantry and punch you in the mouth when you're halfway through crushing a whole line of Oreos. They aren't going to always be there to make sure you get to the gym—even when you're on vacation—and then push you once you're there. Your character does that. Your character is the predictor 100% of how you will behave. And you can't half-act your character either. Think of character like an internal motor that has to be firing on all cylinders at all time. When you act in your best interest and with your best character in mind, you might give the Girl Scouts 20 dollars and then politely say, "Take a hike. Make sure those Thin Mints don't end up at my door." It's sitting in a hotel room and deciding a 30-minute workout in their crappy gym, is more important than turning on the TV or taking a nap. Your character should allow positive effects in your life for times when you don't have access to a gym, and your accountability group is hundreds of miles away.

THAT is character.

Fitness journeys are all so different and have different paths, goals, and people, but every one of these journeys ends up at one of two destinations: Success or failure. If you create a solid accountability group, find the necessary support, and ensure that your character is exactly where it needs to be, you will succeed as you strive to hit healthier goals. You will be better. You will live a longer, happier, healthier life.

So, take the metaphorical or literal punch to the mouth; take the help from the people who love you, and make sure that every day you are relentlessly and passionately pursuing happiness. When you do this, you will be one successful mother trucker.

Time

The most common excuse for not exercising is not having the time. It is extremely difficult to make time for exercise when you have so many other obligations in your life. We all say, "I'd love to exercise more, but I have to work. I have to take the kids to practice. I travel too much," and so on. Time is a valuable commodity, the ultimate limited resource. Whether you like it or not, exercise has to become a part of your life even in the midst of this limited resource. Every day, more and more research reveals that living a sedentary lifestyle is a major contributor to heart disease, diabetes, and obesity. The Centers for Disease Control and Prevention (CDC) recommends 150 to 300 minutes of moderate-intensity activity each week to attain the most health benefits. The demands of family, work, and social life taking a toll on your schedule leads you to weed out tasks that seem unimportant. If physical activity has fallen into that category, it is time to re-evaluate your priorities.

Every day, you are forced to make multiple decisions about what's important to you and what's not, and then you are expected to prioritize accordingly. You decide when to get up in the morning; you decide if you're going to work; you decide if you're going to walk the dog, feed the kids, or pay your mortgage, etc. Your list may look something like this:

1. Family (pets)
2. Work
3. Sleep

4. Food

5. Entertainment/Relaxation

6. Friends

These priorities are considered "no-brainers." You don't even have to think about them; you just accept and take care of them. Over the years, you learn to prioritize your list because if you don't, you'll be fired, lose your house, your kids will starve, and so on.

Question: So, why isn't exercise on your list?

Answer: Because most people are in denial about their health.

We all have reasons for not exercising, but what we choose to do comes down to time management and fear. Fear of embarrassment. Fear of getting hurt. Fear of failure. What you should be afraid of, however, is what will happen to you if you *don't* exercise. How will your sedentary lifestyle affect you next year, in five years, or 10 years? Will you have time for multiple doctors' appointments? Will you have the time and funds to take medication every day to treat high cholesterol, high blood pressure, or diabetes?

As busy are you are, I assure you, extra minutes are hiding in your day that you could use more effectively. The key to exercising regularly is to make exercise part of your daily routine. In other words, it should feel weird if you miss your workout!

Here are some tips to fit exercise into your busy schedule:

1. Figure out the best time exercise will fit into your current schedule. Enter it into your phone calendar, task reminder, or planner, and then set an alarm.

2. Keep your commute to the gym as short as possible. Find a gym that is close to where you live or work.

3. Bring your gym clothes with you to work or keep them in your car. This is imperative to creating efficiency. Having your gym clothes with you serves as a continual reminder that you made a promise to yourself. Set yourself up for success by packing your bag nightly.

4. When you pick out your clothes, pick out your kid's clothes, too. Pack their bags and lunches ahead of time. Meal prep throughout the week for your entire family.

5. Treat your workout as an appointment that you cannot cancel. The only way to make exercise a part of your daily routine is by forcing yourself to go no matter what.

When you do this, you will create a habit to exercise.

6. Treat exercise like an investment. Why would you invest money into a venture that would only return one percent? Meaning, find a workout routine that targets multiple muscle groups at once. Everyone can carve out 30 minutes from their day to exercise. And when you break it down, that's only 2% of your day!

7. Make it fun! One of the best motivators is to look forward to your training fun. Keep a journal of your progress and aim for small wins every day. Be better than you were the day before (weight increase, sets, reps, etc.) Your only competition is who you were yesterday. Having a workout buddy with you also makes training not only fun but holds you accountable.

8. Work out before your day gets in the way. It is hard for me to get my workout in after work because I'd get tired and make all kinds of excuses. Get it done while the kids are still asleep; no one needs your attention at 5:35am.

9. Make sure that the time you do spend exercising is used as efficiently and effectively as possible. Spend less time exercising by doing High-Intensity Interval Training (HIIT). You not only burn a lot of calories during these workouts, but you will continue to burn calories throughout the day as your body replaces energy and repairs muscle proteins damaged during exercise.

10. Spend your time wisely. Figure out which activities you can take time from in your day: those 15 minutes of checking Facebook

or 20 minutes aimlessly surfing the TV or internet—add them up and use them for the gym.

11. Delegate your housework. Just admit it, you can't do it all! Maybe your kids can clean or tidy up the house, or your spouse can cook dinner. Maybe chores can be done less often, or a particular task might not need to be done at all...yet. You just have to "let it go" sometimes.

12. Most of all, don't beat yourself up. Life happens in different forms: sick days, family functions, school and sporting events, etc. Sometimes, you just need that extra time to spend with your family. Give yourself grace, and then try again. As long as you're doing your best every day, you will eventually reach your goals.

I challenge you to use these tips to fit an exercise session into your daily routine. At Platinum Fitness, our 30-minute HIIT classes are perfect for those with a busy schedule. We offer 13 sessions daily to accommodate every clients' needs. We help you maximize your time by focusing on major muscle groups. There is no guesswork as certified personal trainers lead each class. It is also a blast! And that is a critical ingredient in your workout. It can't feel like drudgery! A group setting is a great way for you to work out with friends or meet new people.

No matter what, no one (including us) can force you to take that path to a healthier you. You can keep putting everything and everyone else before you, or you can choose to become a better version of you. You can keep feeding your body junk, or you can start eating right. The former means a life likely full of illness, injuries and pain. The latter steers you toward a life of happiness, adventure, and independence as you age.

The obvious answer is to start making exercise a part of your priority list right now. So, what will you choose?

Self-care is hard but possible. More importantly, it's necessary! You can't care for your family if you don't take care of yourself first. It's time to figure out how to fit some "ME" time into your day. You owe yourself that much!

We're here to support you no matter what your journey looks like, and what your needs are.

Platinum Fitness operates on the concept of serving you first, making you comfortable, and building your accountability team as you are supported in reaching every fitness goal you have always longed for.

About the Author

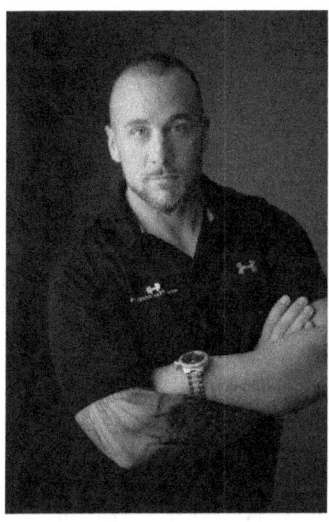

Aaron Nash is the multi-award-winning gym owner of Platinum Fitness, LLC, one of the fastest growing 7-figure fitness centers in the United States. He combines the unique experience of group HIIT training workouts, fat loss nutrition programs, and mindset coaching to lead clients to their healthiest results.

Formerly from West Michigan, Aaron now lives in South Florida. He has helped over 150 people lose more than 50 lbs. in five years, equaling a grand total of over 200,000 client lbs. lost. While Aaron and his highly-trained staff mentor clients in elevating their mindset, they emphasize implementing the formula to success first in one area of their lives before applying it to other aspects. His method creates consistent, abundant, and balanced lives clients can maintain as they continually challenge themselves.

When Aaron is not running his fitness powerhouses, he enjoys spending time with his wife and kiddo and playing with his bulldogs.